HIGH BLOOD

PRESSURE

COOKBOOK

DR. MAUREEN MOORE

TABLE OF CONTENT

CHAPTER ONE

Introduction

Welcome to the "Delicious Recipes for Managing High Blood Pressure". This comprehensive cookbook is designed to support individuals who are navigating the journey of managing high blood pressure through dietary adjustments. High blood pressure, or hypertension, is a common condition that affects millions of people worldwide and is often referred to as the "silent killer" due to its subtle symptoms and serious health implications.

In this cookbook, we have curated a collection of flavorful, heart-healthy recipes that prioritize ingredients known to promote lower blood pressure and overall cardiovascular health. Each recipe is carefully crafted to be low in sodium, saturated fats, and refined sugars while incorporating nutrient-rich foods such as fruits, vegetables, lean proteins, whole grains, and heart-healthy fats.

Managing high blood pressure through dietary modifications is a key aspect of maintaining cardiovascular health and reducing the risk of complications such as heart disease, stroke, and kidney damage. By making smart food choices and adopting a balanced eating pattern, individuals can significantly improve their blood pressure levels and overall well-being.

Whether you're newly diagnosed with high blood pressure or have been managing it for years, this cookbook serves as a valuable resource for creating delicious and nourishing meals that support your heart health goals. From vibrant salads and satisfying soups to flavorful mains and wholesome snacks, each recipe is designed to inspire you to embrace a heart-healthy lifestyle without sacrificing flavor or enjoyment.

In addition to mouthwatering recipes, this cookbook also provides practical tips for grocery shopping, meal planning, and dining out, as well as helpful information on understanding nutrition labels and portion control. With the right tools and resources at your fingertips, you can take control of your health and embark on a journey towards better blood pressure management and improved overall health.

Whether you're cooking for yourself, your family, or entertaining guests, the "Healthy Hearts Cookbook" is your ultimate guide to delicious, heart-healthy eating that nourishes your body and supports your journey to optimal health. Let's embark on this culinary adventure together and take proactive steps towards a healthier, happier heart!

Understanding High Blood Pressure Cookbook:

Welcome to the "Understanding High Blood Pressure Cookbook: Delicious Recipes for Managing Hypertension". This cookbook is your comprehensive guide to navigating the dietary aspects of managing high blood pressure, also known as hypertension. With millions of individuals affected by this condition worldwide, it's crucial to adopt a heart-healthy diet to support overall well-being and reduce the risk of complications.

Understanding the Importance of Diet in Managing High Blood Pressure:

Diet plays a pivotal role in managing high blood pressure. By making mindful choices about the foods we eat, we can positively impact our blood pressure levels and overall cardiovascular health. The recipes in this cookbook are thoughtfully crafted to be low in sodium, saturated fats, and refined sugars while being rich in essential nutrients like potassium, magnesium, and fiber, which are known to support healthy blood pressure.

Navigating the Journey of Hypertension:

Managing high blood pressure can feel overwhelming, but it's essential to approach it with knowledge and empowerment. This cookbook aims to provide you with the tools and resources you need to take control of your health through delicious and nourishing meals. From vibrant salads to comforting soups and hearty mains, each recipe is designed to be flavorful, satisfying, and heart-healthy.

Key Features of the Cookbook:

Mouthwatering Recipes: Explore a diverse array of recipes that cater to different tastes and preferences while prioritizing heart-healthy ingredients.

Nutritional Information: Each recipe is accompanied by nutritional information, making it easier for you to track your intake of key nutrients and make informed food choices.

Practical Tips and Guidance: In addition to recipes, this cookbook offers practical tips and guidance on meal planning, grocery shopping, dining out, and understanding nutrition labels.

Empowerment and Support: Managing high blood pressure is a journey, and this cookbook aims to empower you with the knowledge and resources you need to succeed. Whether you're cooking for yourself or your loved ones, you'll find inspiration and support within these pages.

Embark on a journey towards better health and well-being with the "Understanding High Blood Pressure Cookbook". By embracing a heart-healthy diet and making positive lifestyle changes, you can take control of your blood pressure and enjoy a fulfilling and vibrant life. Let this cookbook be your guide to delicious, nutritious eating that nourishes your body and supports your journey to optimal health.

Principles of High Blood Pressure Cookbook:

Welcome to the "Principles of High Blood Pressure Cookbook: Nourishing Recipes for Heart Health". This cookbook is designed to provide you with a comprehensive understanding of the principles behind managing high blood pressure through dietary interventions.

High blood pressure, or hypertension, is a prevalent condition that requires proactive management to reduce the risk of complications such as heart disease, stroke, and kidney damage.

Principle 1: Mindful Sodium Reduction

One of the fundamental principles of managing high blood pressure is reducing sodium intake. Excessive sodium consumption can contribute to elevated blood pressure levels. Therefore, the recipes in this cookbook are crafted to be low in sodium while still being flavorful and satisfying. We utilize herbs, spices, and other seasonings to enhance the taste of dishes without relying on salt.

Principle 2: Embracing Heart-Healthy Ingredients

Another key principle is incorporating heart-healthy ingredients into your meals. These include fruits, vegetables, whole grains, lean proteins, and unsaturated fats. These nutrient-rich foods are packed with vitamins, minerals, and antioxidants that support cardiovascular health and help lower blood pressure. Our recipes focus on showcasing these ingredients in delicious and creative ways.

Principle 3: Balancing Macronutrients

Balancing macronutrients—carbohydrates, proteins, and fats—is essential for maintaining stable blood sugar levels and supporting overall health. Our recipes are carefully crafted to provide a balance of these macronutrients, with an emphasis on complex carbohydrates, lean proteins, and healthy fats. This ensures that each meal is satisfying, nourishing, and conducive to managing high blood pressure.

Principle 4: Portion Control and Moderation

Portion control and moderation are crucial aspects of managing high blood pressure. Even healthy foods can contribute to weight gain and elevated blood pressure if consumed in excess. Therefore, our recipes are designed to promote portion awareness and mindful eating. We provide serving sizes and nutritional information to help you make informed choices and maintain a healthy balance.

Principle 5: Sustainability and Enjoyment

Finally, sustainability and enjoyment are essential principles of any dietary approach. Sustainable dietary habits are ones that you can maintain over the long term, leading to lasting improvements in health outcomes. Likewise, enjoyment is key to adherence and satisfaction with your dietary choices. Our recipes are designed to be both sustainable and enjoyable, ensuring that you can maintain a healthy lifestyle without feeling deprived.

By embracing the principles outlined in this cookbook, you can take proactive steps towards managing your high blood pressure and improving your overall health and well-being. Through mindful sodium reduction, embracing heart-healthy ingredients, balancing macronutrients, practicing portion control and moderation, and prioritizing sustainability and enjoyment, you can create delicious and nourishing meals that support your journey to optimal health. Let this cookbook be your guide to nourishing your body, nurturing your heart, and enjoying a vibrant and fulfilling life.

Benefits of High Blood Pressure Cookbook:

The "Benefits of High Blood Pressure Cookbook" is more than just a collection of recipes—it's a comprehensive guide to improving your overall health and well-being by managing hypertension through dietary interventions. High blood pressure, or hypertension, affects millions of individuals worldwide and is a significant risk factor for cardiovascular disease. However, by making smart food choices and adopting a heart-healthy eating pattern, you can significantly reduce your risk of complications and improve your quality of life.

Benefit 1: Heart-Healthy Recipes

One of the primary benefits of this cookbook is its focus on heart-healthy recipes. Each recipe is carefully crafted to be low in sodium, saturated fats, and refined sugars while incorporating nutrient-rich ingredients that support cardiovascular health. From vibrant salads and satisfying soups to flavorful mains and wholesome snacks, these recipes are designed to nourish your body and nurture your heart.

Benefit 2: Lower Blood Pressure Levels

By following the dietary recommendations outlined in this cookbook, you can expect to see improvements in your blood pressure levels over time. Many of the ingredients featured in these recipes, such as fruits, vegetables, whole grains, and lean proteins, are known to have blood pressure-lowering effects. Additionally, reducing sodium intake and focusing on balanced meals can help regulate blood pressure and promote overall cardiovascular health.

Benefit 3: Improved Overall Health

Managing high blood pressure through dietary modifications can have far-reaching benefits beyond just blood pressure control. A heart-healthy diet is associated with a reduced risk of other chronic conditions such as heart disease, stroke, diabetes, and obesity. By prioritizing nutritious, whole foods and minimizing the consumption of processed and unhealthy foods, you can improve your overall health and well-being.

Benefit 4: Delicious and Satisfying Meals

One of the most significant benefits of this cookbook is that it proves that healthy eating doesn't have to be bland or boring. The recipes featured here are flavorful, satisfying, and enjoyable to eat. Whether you're cooking for yourself, your family, or entertaining guests, you can feel confident that the meals you prepare will be both nutritious and delicious.

Benefit 5: Empowerment and Support

Finally, this cookbook provides you with the knowledge, tools, and resources you need to take control of your health and well-being. By empowering you with practical tips, guidance, and delicious recipes, it supports you on your journey to better health. Whether you're newly diagnosed with high blood pressure or have been managing it for years, this cookbook is your trusted companion every step of the way.

The "Benefits of High Blood Pressure Cookbook" offers a wealth of benefits for anyone looking to improve their cardiovascular health and manage hypertension through dietary interventions. From heart-healthy recipes and lower blood pressure levels to improved overall health, delicious meals, and empowerment and support, this cookbook is your ultimate guide to nourishing your body, nurturing your heart, and living your best life. Let this cookbook be your roadmap to better health and well-being—one delicious meal at a time.

Guidelines for High Blood Pressure Cookbook:

The "Guidelines for High Blood Pressure Cookbook" provide you with essential principles and strategies for managing hypertension through dietary interventions. High blood pressure, or hypertension, is a prevalent condition that requires proactive management to reduce the risk of complications and promote overall cardiovascular health. By following these guidelines, you can make informed food choices and adopt a heart-healthy eating pattern that supports your blood pressure management goals.

Guideline 1: Limit Sodium Intake

One of the most critical guidelines for managing high blood pressure is to limit sodium intake. Excessive sodium consumption can contribute to elevated blood pressure levels. Therefore, aim to reduce your sodium intake by choosing fresh, whole foods over processed and packaged foods, which are often high in sodium. Use herbs, spices, and other flavorings to enhance the taste of your meals without relying on salt.

Guideline 2: Emphasize Fruits and Vegetables

Fruits and vegetables are rich in vitamins, minerals, antioxidants, and dietary fiber, making them essential components of a heart-healthy diet. Aim to include a variety of colorful fruits and vegetables in your meals and snacks each day. These nutrient-rich foods help lower blood pressure, improve blood vessel function, and reduce the risk of cardiovascular disease.

Guideline 3: Choose Whole Grains

Whole grains are another essential component of a heart-healthy diet. Unlike refined grains, which have been stripped of their nutrient-rich bran and germ layers, whole grains retain all of their natural fiber, vitamins, and minerals. Choose whole grain options such as brown rice, quinoa, oats, barley, and whole wheat bread and pasta to provide lasting energy and promote satiety.

Guideline 4: Opt for Lean Proteins

Lean proteins are an important part of a heart-healthy diet. Choose lean protein sources such as skinless poultry, fish, seafood, beans, lentils, tofu, and low-fat dairy products. These protein-rich foods provide essential nutrients without the saturated fats found in fatty cuts of meat and processed meats, which can raise cholesterol levels and increase the risk of heart disease.

Guideline 5: Limit Saturated and Trans Fats

Saturated and trans fats are unhealthy fats that can raise cholesterol levels and increase the risk of heart disease. Limit your intake of foods high in saturated and trans fats, such as fatty meats, full-fat dairy products, butter, margarine, and processed foods. Instead, choose heart-healthy fats such as olive oil, avocado, nuts, seeds, and fatty fish, which provide essential omega-3 fatty acids and support cardiovascular health.

Guideline 6: Practice Portion Control

Portion control is essential for managing high blood pressure and maintaining a healthy weight. Be mindful of portion sizes and avoid oversized servings, which can lead to excess calorie intake and weight gain. Use smaller plates and bowls, measure out serving sizes, and pay attention to hunger and fullness cues to prevent overeating.

Guideline 7: Stay Hydrated

Staying hydrated is crucial for overall health and well-being, including blood pressure regulation. Aim to drink plenty of water throughout the day and limit your intake of sugary beverages, caffeinated drinks, and alcohol, which can dehydrate the body and affect blood pressure levels. Drinking water helps flush out toxins, supports healthy blood circulation, and keeps your body functioning optimally.

Guideline 8: Practice Mindful Eating

Finally, practice mindful eating to cultivate a healthy relationship with food and promote better blood pressure management. Pay attention to hunger and fullness cues, eat slowly and mindfully, and savor each bite. Avoid distractions such as television, smartphones, and computers while eating, as these can lead to mindless overeating and poor food choices.

By following these guidelines for managing high blood pressure, you can make informed food choices and adopt a heart-healthy eating pattern that supports your blood pressure management goals. By prioritizing low-sodium, nutrient-rich foods such as fruits, vegetables, whole grains, lean proteins, and healthy fats, and practicing portion control and mindful eating, you can take proactive steps towards better health and well-being. Let these guidelines be your roadmap to managing high blood pressure and living a heart-healthy lifestyle.

Recipe 1: Heart-Healthy Spinach and Avocado Salad

Ingredients:

4 cups fresh spinach leaves

1 ripe avocado, diced

1/2 cup cherry tomatoes, halved

1/4 cup red onion, thinly sliced

2 tablespoons extra virgin olive oil

1 tablespoon balsamic vinegar

1 teaspoon Dijon mustard

Salt and pepper to taste

Optional: crumbled feta cheese or toasted nuts for garnish

Instructions:

In a large mixing bowl, combine the fresh spinach leaves, diced avocado, halved cherry tomatoes, and thinly sliced red onion.

In a small bowl, whisk together the extra virgin olive oil, balsamic vinegar, and Dijon mustard to make the dressing.

Drizzle the dressing over the salad ingredients and toss gently to coat.

Season with salt and pepper to taste.

Optional: Sprinkle crumbled feta cheese or toasted nuts over the top for added flavor and texture.

Serve immediately as a refreshing and nutritious side dish or light meal.

Benefits:

This heart-healthy spinach and avocado salad is packed with nutrient-rich ingredients that support cardiovascular health.

Spinach is high in potassium and magnesium, which help regulate blood pressure levels.

Avocado provides heart-healthy monounsaturated fats and potassium, which may help lower blood pressure.

Cherry tomatoes are rich in antioxidants such as lycopene, which may have protective effects on the cardiovascular system.

Cooking Time: 10 minutes

Recipe 2: Garlic Herb Baked Salmon

Ingredients:

4 salmon fillets (about 6 ounces each)

2 tablespoons extra virgin olive oil

2 cloves garlic, minced

1 tablespoon fresh lemon juice

1 teaspoon dried thyme

1 teaspoon dried rosemary

Salt and pepper to taste

Lemon wedges for serving

Instructions:

Preheat the oven to 400°F (200°C). Line a baking sheet with parchment paper.

Place the salmon fillets on the prepared baking sheet.

In a small bowl, whisk together the extra virgin olive oil, minced garlic, fresh lemon juice, dried thyme, dried rosemary, salt, and pepper.

Drizzle the garlic herb mixture over the salmon fillets, ensuring they are evenly coated.

Bake in the preheated oven for 12-15 minutes, or until the salmon is cooked through and flakes easily with a fork.

Remove from the oven and let rest for a few minutes before serving.

Serve hot with lemon wedges on the side for squeezing over the salmon.

Benefits:

This garlic herb baked salmon is a flavorful and nutritious dish that is rich in omega-3 fatty acids, which support heart health.

Salmon is an excellent source of protein and contains beneficial nutrients such as vitamin D and selenium.

Garlic has been shown to have potential blood pressure-lowering effects and may help improve cardiovascular health.

Herbs such as thyme and rosemary add aromatic flavor and provide antioxidant properties.

Cooking Time: 15 minutes

Recipe 3: Quinoa and Vegetable Stir-Fry

Ingredients:

1 cup quinoa, rinsed and drained

2 cups water or low-sodium vegetable broth

1 tablespoon sesame oil

2 cloves garlic, minced

1 tablespoon grated ginger

1 bell pepper, thinly sliced

1 cup broccoli florets

1 cup snap peas, trimmed

1 carrot, julienned

2 tablespoons low-sodium soy sauce or tamari

1 tablespoon rice vinegar

1 teaspoon honey or maple syrup (optional)

Sesame seeds for garnish (optional)

Chopped green onions for garnish (optional)

Instructions:

In a medium saucepan, combine the rinsed quinoa and water or vegetable broth. Bring to a boil, then reduce the heat to low, cover, and simmer for 15-20 minutes, or until the quinoa is tender and the liquid is absorbed. Remove from heat and let stand for 5 minutes before fluffing with a fork.

In a large skillet or wok, heat the sesame oil over medium heat. Add the minced garlic and grated ginger, and cook for 1-2 minutes until fragrant.

Add the thinly sliced bell pepper, broccoli florets, snap peas, and julienned carrot to the skillet. Stir-fry for 5-7 minutes, or until the vegetables are tender-crisp.

In a small bowl, whisk together the low-sodium soy sauce or tamari, rice vinegar, and honey or maple syrup (if using).

Add the cooked quinoa to the skillet with the stir-fried vegetables, and pour the sauce over the top. Stir to combine and heat through.

Garnish with sesame seeds and chopped green onions, if desired.

Serve hot as a nutritious and satisfying main dish or side dish.

Benefits:

This quinoa and vegetable stir-fry is a nutrient-rich dish that provides a balance of complex carbohydrates, protein, fiber, vitamins, and minerals.

Quinoa is a complete protein source and contains heart-healthy nutrients such as potassium and magnesium.

Colorful vegetables like bell pepper, broccoli, snap peas, and carrot provide essential vitamins, minerals, and antioxidants that support cardiovascular health.

Sesame oil and sesame seeds add a rich, nutty flavor and provide heart-healthy unsaturated fats.

Cooking Time: 30 minutes

Recipe 4: Grilled Lemon Herb Chicken

Ingredients:

4 boneless, skinless chicken breasts

2 tablespoons extra virgin olive oil

2 tablespoons fresh lemon juice

2 cloves garlic, minced

1 tablespoon chopped fresh herbs (such as parsley, thyme, or rosemary)

Salt and pepper to taste

Lemon slices for garnish

Instructions:

In a small bowl, whisk together the extra virgin olive oil, fresh lemon juice, minced garlic, chopped fresh herbs, salt, and pepper to make the marinade.

Place the chicken breasts in a shallow dish or resealable plastic bag. Pour the marinade over the chicken, ensuring it is evenly coated. Marinate in the refrigerator for at least 30 minutes, or up to 4 hours.

Preheat grill to medium-high heat. Remove the chicken from the marinade and discard any excess marinade.

Grill the chicken breasts for 6-8 minutes per side, or until cooked through and no longer pink in the center.

Remove from the grill and let rest for a few minutes before serving.

Garnish with lemon slices before serving.

Benefits:

This grilled lemon herb chicken is a lean protein option that is low in saturated fat and cholesterol, making it heart-healthy.

Fresh lemon juice adds a burst of citrus flavor and provides vitamin C, which is essential for immune health and may help lower blood pressure.

Garlic and fresh herbs not only enhance the flavor of the chicken but also provide antioxidant properties that support cardiovascular health.

Cooking Time: 20 minutes (plus marinating time)

Recipe 5: Mediterranean Stuffed Bell Peppers

Ingredients:

4 large bell peppers (any color)

1 cup cooked quinoa

1 cup diced tomatoes

1/2 cup chopped cucumber

1/4 cup chopped Kalamata olives

1/4 cup crumbled feta cheese

2 tablespoons chopped fresh parsley

1 tablespoon extra virgin olive oil

1 tablespoon lemon juice

2 cloves garlic, minced

1 teaspoon dried oregano

Salt and pepper to taste

Instructions:

Preheat oven to 375°F (190°C). Cut the tops off the bell peppers and remove the seeds and membranes. Place the bell peppers upright in a baking dish.

In a mixing bowl, combine cooked quinoa, diced tomatoes, chopped cucumber, Kalamata olives, crumbled feta cheese, chopped fresh parsley, extra virgin olive oil, lemon juice, minced garlic, dried oregano, salt, and pepper. Mix well to combine.

Stuff each bell pepper with the quinoa mixture until they are filled to the top.

Cover the baking dish with aluminum foil and bake in the preheated oven for 30-35 minutes, or until the bell peppers are tender.

Remove from the oven and let cool for a few minutes before serving.

Garnish with additional chopped parsley if desired.

Benefits:

These Mediterranean stuffed bell peppers are packed with heart-healthy ingredients such as quinoa, tomatoes, cucumber, olives, and olive oil.

Quinoa provides a complete source of protein and essential nutrients like fiber, potassium, and magnesium, which support cardiovascular health.

The combination of fresh vegetables, herbs, and olive oil adds vibrant flavors and provides a variety of vitamins, minerals, and antioxidants that promote heart health.

Cooking Time: 40 minutes

Recipe 6: Garlic Lemon Shrimp and Broccoli Stir-Fry

Ingredients:

1 lb large shrimp, peeled and deveined

4 cups broccoli florets

2 tablespoons extra virgin olive oil

4 cloves garlic, minced

2 tablespoons fresh lemon juice

1 teaspoon lemon zest

1/4 teaspoon red pepper flakes (optional)

Salt and pepper to taste

Chopped fresh parsley for garnish (optional)

Cooked brown rice or quinoa for serving

Instructions:

In a large skillet or wok, heat the extra virgin olive oil over medium-high heat. Add the minced garlic and red pepper flakes (if using), and cook for 1-2 minutes until fragrant.

Add the shrimp to the skillet and cook for 2-3 minutes per side, or until pink and opaque.

Remove the cooked shrimp from the skillet and set aside.

In the same skillet, add the broccoli florets and cook for 4-5 minutes, or until tender-crisp.

Return the cooked shrimp to the skillet with the broccoli.

Add the fresh lemon juice and lemon zest to the skillet, and toss to coat the shrimp and broccoli evenly.

Season with salt and pepper to taste.

Garnish with chopped fresh parsley before serving.

Serve hot with cooked brown rice or quinoa.

Benefits:

This garlic lemon shrimp and broccoli stir-fry is a quick and nutritious dish that is rich in protein, fiber, vitamins, and minerals.

Shrimp is a lean protein source that is low in saturated fat and cholesterol, making it heart-healthy.

Broccoli is packed with antioxidants, fiber, and vitamin C, which support cardiovascular health and help lower blood pressure.

Cooking Time: 20 minutes

Recipe 7: Balsamic Glazed Salmon

Ingredients:

4 salmon fillets (about 6 ounces each)

1/4 cup balsamic vinegar

2 tablespoons honey or maple syrup

2 cloves garlic, minced

1 tablespoon extra virgin olive oil

Salt and pepper to taste

Fresh parsley for garnish (optional)

Instructions:

In a small saucepan, combine the balsamic vinegar, honey or maple syrup, and minced garlic. Bring to a simmer over medium heat and cook for 3-4 minutes, or until the mixture has thickened slightly.

Remove from heat and set aside.

Season the salmon fillets with salt and pepper on both sides.

In a large skillet, heat the extra virgin olive oil over medium-high heat. Add the salmon fillets to the skillet, skin-side down, and cook for 3-4 minutes.

Carefully flip the salmon fillets and brush the tops with the balsamic glaze.

Continue cooking for another 3-4 minutes, or until the salmon is cooked through and flakes easily with a fork.

Remove from heat and drizzle any remaining glaze over the salmon.

Garnish with fresh parsley before serving.

Benefits:

This balsamic glazed salmon is a flavorful and nutritious dish that is rich in omega-3 fatty acids, protein, and essential nutrients.

Balsamic vinegar adds a sweet and tangy flavor to the salmon and provides antioxidants that support heart health.

Honey or maple syrup adds natural sweetness without refined sugars, making this dish suitable for those watching their sugar intake.

Cooking Time: 15 minutes

Recipe 8: Lemon Garlic Roasted Brussels Sprouts

Ingredients:

1 lb Brussels sprouts, trimmed and halved

2 tablespoons extra virgin olive oil

2 cloves garlic, minced

2 tablespoons fresh lemon juice

1 teaspoon lemon zest

Salt and pepper to taste

Grated Parmesan cheese for garnish (optional)

Instructions:

Preheat oven to 400°F (200°C). Line a baking sheet with parchment paper.

In a large mixing bowl, toss the halved Brussels sprouts with extra virgin olive oil, minced garlic, fresh lemon juice, lemon zest, salt, and pepper until evenly coated.

Spread the Brussels sprouts in a single layer on the prepared baking sheet.

Roast in the preheated oven for 20-25 minutes, or until the Brussels sprouts are golden brown and tender, stirring halfway through.

Remove from the oven and transfer to a serving dish.

Garnish with grated Parmesan cheese before serving, if desired.

Benefits:

These lemon garlic roasted Brussels sprouts are a delicious and nutritious side dish that is rich in fiber, vitamins, and minerals.

Brussels sprouts are a cruciferous vegetable that provides antioxidants and anti-inflammatory properties that support heart health.

Garlic and lemon add aromatic flavor and provide additional heart-healthy benefits, including potential blood pressure-lowering effects.

Cooking Time: 25 minutes

Recipe 9: Turkey and Vegetable Skillet

Ingredients:

1 lb ground turkey

1 tablespoon extra virgin olive oil

1 onion, diced

2 cloves garlic, minced

1 bell pepper, diced

1 zucchini, diced

1 cup cherry tomatoes, halved

1 teaspoon dried oregano

1 teaspoon dried basil

Salt and pepper to taste

Fresh parsley for garnish (optional)

Instructions:

In a large skillet, heat the extra virgin olive oil over medium heat. Add the diced onion and minced garlic, and cook for 2-3 minutes until softened and fragrant.

Add the ground turkey to the skillet and cook, breaking it apart with a spatula, until browned and cooked through.

Add the diced bell pepper and zucchini to the skillet, and cook for an additional 5-7 minutes, or until the vegetables are tender.

Stir in the halved cherry tomatoes, dried oregano, and dried basil. Cook for another 2-3 minutes to heat through.

Season with salt and pepper to taste.

Garnish with fresh parsley before serving.

Benefits:

This turkey and vegetable skillet is a quick and easy one-pan meal that is high in protein, fiber, vitamins, and minerals.

Ground turkey is a lean protein source that is lower in saturated fat than red meat, making it heart-healthy.

Colorful vegetables like bell pepper, zucchini, and cherry tomatoes provide antioxidants and essential nutrients that support cardiovascular health.

Cooking Time: 25 minutes

Recipe 10: Mediterranean Chickpea Salad

Ingredients:

2 cups cooked chickpeas (canned or cooked from dry)

1 cucumber, diced

1 bell pepper, diced

1/2 red onion, thinly sliced

1 cup cherry tomatoes, halved

1/4 cup Kalamata olives, sliced

1/4 cup crumbled feta cheese

2 tablespoons chopped fresh parsley

2 tablespoons extra virgin olive oil

1 tablespoon red wine vinegar

1 teaspoon dried oregano

Salt and pepper to taste

Lemon wedges for serving (optional)

Instructions:

In a large mixing bowl, combine the cooked chickpeas, diced cucumber, diced bell pepper, thinly sliced red onion, halved cherry tomatoes, sliced Kalamata olives, crumbled feta cheese, and chopped fresh parsley.

In a small bowl, whisk together the extra virgin olive oil, red wine vinegar, dried oregano, salt, and pepper to make the dressing.

Pour the dressing over the chickpea salad ingredients and toss gently to coat.

Serve the Mediterranean chickpea salad immediately, or refrigerate for 30 minutes to allow the flavors to meld.

Garnish with lemon wedges before serving, if desired.

Benefits:

This Mediterranean chickpea salad is a refreshing and nutritious dish that is high in fiber, protein, vitamins, and minerals.

Chickpeas are rich in soluble fiber, which may help lower cholesterol levels and improve heart health.

Colorful vegetables like cucumber, bell pepper, red onion, and cherry tomatoes provide antioxidants and essential nutrients that support cardiovascular health.

Olive oil and feta cheese provide heart-healthy monounsaturated fats and calcium, respectively.

Cooking Time: 15 minutes

Recipe 11: Lemon Herb Grilled Chicken

Ingredients:

4 boneless, skinless chicken breasts

1/4 cup fresh lemon juice

2 tablespoons extra virgin olive oil

2 cloves garlic, minced

2 teaspoons chopped fresh thyme

2 teaspoons chopped fresh rosemary

Salt and pepper to taste

Lemon slices for garnish

Instructions:

In a small bowl, whisk together the fresh lemon juice, extra virgin olive oil, minced garlic, chopped fresh thyme, chopped fresh rosemary, salt, and pepper to make the marinade.

Place the chicken breasts in a shallow dish or resealable plastic bag. Pour the marinade over the chicken, ensuring it is evenly coated. Marinate in the refrigerator for at least 30 minutes, or up to 4 hours.

Preheat grill to medium-high heat. Remove the chicken from the marinade and discard any excess marinade.

Grill the chicken breasts for 6-8 minutes per side, or until cooked through and no longer pink in the center.

Remove from the grill and let rest for a few minutes before serving.

Garnish with lemon slices before serving.

Benefits:

This lemon herb grilled chicken is a lean protein option that is low in saturated fat and cholesterol, making it heart-healthy.

Fresh lemon juice provides a burst of citrus flavor and adds vitamin C, which supports immune health and may help lower blood pressure.

Garlic and fresh herbs like thyme and rosemary not only enhance the flavor of the chicken but also provide antioxidant properties that support cardiovascular health.

Cooking Time: 20 minutes (plus marinating time)

Recipe 12: Quinoa and Black Bean Stuffed Peppers

Ingredients:

4 large bell peppers (any color)

1 cup cooked quinoa

1 cup cooked black beans (canned or cooked from dry)

1 cup diced tomatoes

1/2 cup corn kernels (fresh, frozen, or canned)

1/4 cup chopped fresh cilantro

1 teaspoon ground cumin

1 teaspoon chili powder

Salt and pepper to taste

Grated cheddar cheese for topping (optional)

Sliced avocado for serving (optional)

Instructions:

Preheat oven to 375°F (190°C). Cut the tops off the bell peppers and remove the seeds and membranes. Place the bell peppers upright in a baking dish.

In a mixing bowl, combine the cooked quinoa, cooked black beans, diced tomatoes, corn kernels, chopped fresh cilantro, ground cumin, chili powder, salt, and pepper.

Stuff each bell pepper with the quinoa and black bean mixture until they are filled to the top.

Cover the baking dish with aluminum foil and bake in the preheated oven for 30-35 minutes, or until the bell peppers are tender.

Remove from the oven and sprinkle grated cheddar cheese over the top of each stuffed pepper, if desired. Return to the oven for 5 minutes, or until the cheese is melted and bubbly.

Serve hot with sliced avocado on the side, if desired.

Benefits:

These quinoa and black bean stuffed peppers are a nutritious and satisfying dish that is high in protein, fiber, vitamins, and minerals.

Quinoa provides a complete source of protein and essential nutrients like fiber, potassium, and magnesium, which support cardiovascular health.

Black beans are rich in fiber and plant-based protein, which help lower cholesterol levels and improve heart health.

Colorful vegetables like diced tomatoes, corn kernels, and bell peppers provide antioxidants and essential nutrients that support cardiovascular health.

Cooking Time: 45 minutes

Recipe 13: Garlic Herb Roasted Cauliflower

Ingredients:

1 head cauliflower, cut into florets

2 tablespoons extra virgin olive oil

4 cloves garlic, minced

1 teaspoon dried thyme

1 teaspoon dried rosemary

Salt and pepper to taste

Fresh parsley for garnish (optional)

Lemon wedges for serving (optional)

Instructions:

Preheat oven to 400°F (200°C). Line a baking sheet with parchment paper.

In a large mixing bowl, toss the cauliflower florets with extra virgin olive oil, minced garlic, dried thyme, dried rosemary, salt, and pepper until evenly coated.

Spread the cauliflower in a single layer on the prepared baking sheet.

Roast in the preheated oven for 25-30 minutes, or until the cauliflower is golden brown and tender, stirring halfway through.

Remove from the oven and transfer to a serving dish.

Garnish with fresh parsley and serve hot with lemon wedges on the side, if desired.

Benefits:

This garlic herb roasted cauliflower is a flavorful and nutritious side dish that is low in calories and carbohydrates.

Cauliflower is rich in antioxidants and fiber, which support heart health and may help lower cholesterol levels.

Garlic and herbs like thyme and rosemary add aromatic flavor and provide additional heart-healthy benefits, including potential blood pressure-lowering effects.

Cooking Time: 30 minutes

Recipe 14: Turkey and Spinach Meatballs

Ingredients:

1 lb ground turkey

1 cup fresh spinach, finely chopped

1/4 cup grated Parmesan cheese

1/4 cup breadcrumbs (gluten-free if desired)

1 egg

2 cloves garlic, minced

1 teaspoon dried oregano

1 teaspoon dried basil

Salt and pepper to taste

Olive oil for cooking

Instructions:

In a large mixing bowl, combine the ground turkey, chopped fresh spinach, grated Parmesan cheese, breadcrumbs, egg, minced garlic, dried oregano, dried basil, salt, and pepper. Mix until well combined.

Shape the mixture into meatballs, about 1 inch in diameter.

In a large skillet, heat olive oil over medium heat. Add the meatballs to the skillet, ensuring they are not overcrowded.

Cook the meatballs for 8-10 minutes, turning occasionally, until browned on all sides and cooked through.

Remove from the skillet and drain on paper towels to remove excess oil.

Serve the turkey and spinach meatballs hot with your favorite sauce or as a topping for salads or pasta.

Benefits:

These turkey and spinach meatballs are a lean protein option that is low in saturated fat and cholesterol, making them heart-healthy.

Spinach is rich in vitamins, minerals, and antioxidants that support heart health and may help lower blood pressure.

Using ground turkey instead of beef reduces the overall fat content of the meatballs while still providing essential nutrients like protein and iron.

Cooking Time: 20 minutes

Recipe 15: Lemon Garlic Roasted Asparagus

Ingredients:

1 lb asparagus spears, trimmed

2 tablespoons extra virgin olive oil

4 cloves garlic, minced

2 tablespoons fresh lemon juice

1 teaspoon lemon zest

Salt and pepper to taste

Grated Parmesan cheese for garnish (optional)

Instructions:

Preheat oven to 400°F (200°C). Line a baking sheet with parchment paper.

Arrange the trimmed asparagus spears in a single layer on the prepared baking sheet.

In a small bowl, whisk together the extra virgin olive oil, minced garlic, fresh lemon juice, lemon zest, salt, and pepper.

Drizzle the lemon garlic mixture over the asparagus spears, tossing to coat evenly.

Roast in the preheated oven for 12-15 minutes, or until the asparagus is tender and lightly browned, shaking the pan halfway through.

Remove from the oven and transfer to a serving dish.

Garnish with grated Parmesan cheese before serving, if desired.

Benefits:

This lemon garlic roasted asparagus is a flavorful and nutritious side dish that is low in calories and carbohydrates.

Asparagus is rich in fiber, vitamins, and antioxidants, which support heart health and may help lower cholesterol levels.

Garlic and lemon add aromatic flavor and provide additional heart-healthy benefits, including potential blood pressure-lowering effects.

Cooking Time: 15 minutes

Recipe 16: Greek Quinoa Salad

Ingredients:

1 cup cooked quinoa

1 cup cucumber, diced

1 cup cherry tomatoes, halved

1/2 cup Kalamata olives, sliced

1/4 cup red onion, finely chopped

1/4 cup crumbled feta cheese

2 tablespoons chopped fresh parsley

2 tablespoons extra virgin olive oil

1 tablespoon red wine vinegar

1 teaspoon dried oregano

Salt and pepper to taste

Lemon wedges for serving (optional)

Instructions:

In a large mixing bowl, combine the cooked quinoa, diced cucumber, halved cherry tomatoes, sliced Kalamata olives, finely chopped red onion, crumbled feta cheese, and chopped fresh parsley.

In a small bowl, whisk together the extra virgin olive oil, red wine vinegar, dried oregano, salt, and pepper to make the dressing.

Pour the dressing over the quinoa salad ingredients and toss gently to coat.

Serve the Greek quinoa salad immediately, or refrigerate for 30 minutes to allow the flavors to meld.

Garnish with lemon wedges before serving, if desired.

Benefits:

This Greek quinoa salad is a refreshing and nutritious dish that is high in fiber, protein, vitamins, and minerals.

Quinoa provides a complete source of protein and essential nutrients like fiber, potassium, and magnesium, which support cardiovascular health.

Mediterranean ingredients like cucumber, tomatoes, olives, and feta cheese provide antioxidants and heart-healthy monounsaturated fats.

Cooking Time: 15 minutes

Recipe 17: Herb-Roasted Sweet Potatoes

Ingredients:

2 large sweet potatoes, peeled and cut into cubes

2 tablespoons extra virgin olive oil

2 teaspoons dried thyme

2 teaspoons dried rosemary

1 teaspoon garlic powder

Salt and pepper to taste

Chopped fresh parsley for garnish (optional)

Instructions:

Preheat oven to 425°F (220°C). Line a baking sheet with parchment paper.

In a large mixing bowl, toss the sweet potato cubes with extra virgin olive oil, dried thyme, dried rosemary, garlic powder, salt, and pepper until evenly coated.

Spread the seasoned sweet potato cubes in a single layer on the prepared baking sheet.

Roast in the preheated oven for 25-30 minutes, or until the sweet potatoes are tender and caramelized, stirring halfway through.

Remove from the oven and transfer to a serving dish.

Garnish with chopped fresh parsley before serving.

Benefits:

These herb-roasted sweet potatoes are a flavorful and nutritious side dish that is high in fiber, vitamins, and minerals.

Sweet potatoes are rich in beta-carotene, which is converted into vitamin A in the body and supports immune health and vision.

Herbs like thyme and rosemary add aromatic flavor and provide antioxidant properties that support cardiovascular health.

Cooking Time: 30 minutes

Recipe 18: Cucumber Avocado Salad

Ingredients:

2 cucumbers, diced

1 avocado, diced

1/4 cup red onion, thinly sliced

2 tablespoons chopped fresh dill

2 tablespoons chopped fresh parsley

2 tablespoons extra virgin olive oil

1 tablespoon fresh lemon juice

Salt and pepper to taste

Instructions:

In a large mixing bowl, combine the diced cucumbers, diced avocado, thinly sliced red onion, chopped fresh dill, and chopped fresh parsley.

Drizzle the extra virgin olive oil and fresh lemon juice over the cucumber and avocado mixture.

Season with salt and pepper to taste.

Gently toss to coat all the ingredients evenly.

Serve the cucumber avocado salad immediately as a refreshing side dish or light meal.

Benefits:

This cucumber avocado salad is a simple and nutritious dish that is high in fiber, vitamins, and healthy fats.

Cucumbers are hydrating and low in calories, while avocados provide heart-healthy monounsaturated fats and essential nutrients like potassium and vitamin E.

Fresh herbs like dill and parsley add bright flavor and provide antioxidants and anti-inflammatory properties.

Cooking Time: 10 minutes

Recipe 19: Lemon Garlic Roasted Brussels Sprouts

Ingredients:

1 lb Brussels sprouts, trimmed and halved

2 tablespoons extra virgin olive oil

4 cloves garlic, minced

2 tablespoons fresh lemon juice

1 teaspoon lemon zest

Salt and pepper to taste

Grated Parmesan cheese for garnish (optional)

Instructions:

Preheat oven to 400°F (200°C). Line a baking sheet with parchment paper.

In a large mixing bowl, toss the halved Brussels sprouts with extra virgin olive oil, minced garlic, fresh lemon juice, lemon zest, salt, and pepper until evenly coated.

Spread the Brussels sprouts in a single layer on the prepared baking sheet.

Roast in the preheated oven for 25-30 minutes, or until the Brussels sprouts are golden brown and tender, stirring halfway through.

Remove from the oven and transfer to a serving dish.

Garnish with grated Parmesan cheese before serving, if desired.

Benefits:

This lemon garlic roasted Brussels sprouts is a flavorful and nutritious side dish that is low in calories and carbohydrates.

Brussels sprouts are rich in antioxidants and fiber, which support heart health and may help lower cholesterol levels.

Garlic and lemon add aromatic flavor and provide additional heart-healthy benefits, including potential blood pressure-lowering effects.

Cooking Time: 30 minutes

Recipe 20: Turkey and Spinach Meatballs

Ingredients:

1 lb ground turkey

1 cup fresh spinach, finely chopped

1/4 cup grated Parmesan cheese

1/4 cup breadcrumbs (gluten-free if desired)

1 egg

2 cloves garlic, minced

1 teaspoon dried oregano

1 teaspoon dried basil

Salt and pepper to taste

Olive oil for cooking

Instructions:

In a large mixing bowl, combine the ground turkey, chopped fresh spinach, grated Parmesan cheese, breadcrumbs, egg, minced garlic, dried oregano, dried basil, salt, and pepper. Mix until well combined.

Shape the mixture into meatballs, about 1 inch in diameter.

In a large skillet, heat olive oil over medium heat. Add the meatballs to the skillet, ensuring they are not overcrowded.

Cook the meatballs for 8-10 minutes, turning occasionally, until browned on all sides and cooked through.

Remove from the skillet and drain on paper towels to remove excess oil.

Serve the turkey and spinach meatballs hot with your favorite sauce or as a topping for salads or pasta.

Benefits:

These turkey and spinach meatballs are a lean protein option that is low in saturated fat and cholesterol, making them heart-healthy.

Spinach is rich in vitamins, minerals, and antioxidants that support heart health and may help lower blood pressure.

Using ground turkey instead of beef reduces the overall fat content of the meatballs while still providing essential nutrients like protein and iron.

Cooking Time: 20 minutes

Recipe 21: Grilled Lemon Herb Salmon

Ingredients:

4 salmon fillets (about 6 ounces each)

2 tablespoons fresh lemon juice

2 tablespoons extra virgin olive oil

2 cloves garlic, minced

1 tablespoon chopped fresh dill

1 tablespoon chopped fresh parsley

Salt and pepper to taste

Lemon slices for garnish

Instructions:

In a small bowl, whisk together the fresh lemon juice, extra virgin olive oil, minced garlic, chopped fresh dill, chopped fresh parsley, salt, and pepper to make the marinade.

Place the salmon fillets in a shallow dish or resealable plastic bag. Pour the marinade over the salmon, ensuring they are evenly coated. Marinate in the refrigerator for at least 30 minutes, or up to 4 hours.

Preheat grill to medium-high heat. Remove the salmon from the marinade and discard any excess marinade.

Grill the salmon fillets for 4-5 minutes per side, or until cooked through and flaky.

Remove from the grill and let rest for a few minutes before serving.

Garnish with lemon slices before serving.

Benefits:

This grilled lemon herb salmon is a delicious and nutritious dish that is rich in omega-3 fatty acids, protein, and essential nutrients.

Salmon is a fatty fish that is high in heart-healthy omega-3 fatty acids, which have been shown to reduce inflammation and lower the risk of heart disease.

Fresh lemon juice and herbs like dill and parsley add vibrant flavor and provide additional antioxidant and anti-inflammatory properties.

Cooking Time: 10 minutes (plus marinating time)

Recipe 22: Quinoa and Black Bean Stuffed Zucchini

Ingredients:

4 large zucchini

1 cup cooked quinoa

1 cup cooked black beans (canned or cooked from dry)

1 cup diced tomatoes

1/2 cup corn kernels (fresh, frozen, or canned)

1/4 cup chopped fresh cilantro

1 teaspoon ground cumin

1 teaspoon chili powder

Salt and pepper to taste

Grated cheddar cheese for topping (optional)

Sliced avocado for serving (optional)

Instructions:

Preheat oven to 375°F (190°C). Cut the zucchini in half lengthwise and scoop out the seeds to create a hollow center.

In a mixing bowl, combine the cooked quinoa, cooked black beans, diced tomatoes, corn kernels, chopped fresh cilantro, ground cumin, chili powder, salt, and pepper.

Stuff each zucchini half with the quinoa and black bean mixture until they are filled to the top.

Place the stuffed zucchini halves in a baking dish.

Cover the baking dish with aluminum foil and bake in the preheated oven for 25-30 minutes, or until the zucchini are tender.

Remove from the oven and sprinkle grated cheddar cheese over the top of each stuffed zucchini half, if desired. Return to the oven for 5 minutes, or until the cheese is melted and bubbly.

Serve hot with sliced avocado on the side, if desired.

Benefits:

These quinoa and black bean stuffed zucchini are a nutritious and satisfying dish that is high in protein, fiber, vitamins, and minerals.

Zucchini is low in calories and rich in antioxidants and fiber, which support heart health and may help lower cholesterol levels.

Black beans provide plant-based protein and fiber, which help promote satiety and stabilize blood sugar levels.

Cooking Time: 35 minutes

Recipe 23: Lemon Garlic Shrimp Pasta

Ingredients:

8 oz whole wheat spaghetti or pasta of choice

1 lb large shrimp, peeled and deveined

2 tablespoons extra virgin olive oil

4 cloves garlic, minced

Zest of 1 lemon

Juice of 1 lemon

1/4 teaspoon red pepper flakes

Salt and pepper to taste

Chopped fresh parsley for garnish

Grated Parmesan cheese for serving (optional)

Instructions:

Cook the pasta according to the package instructions until al dente. Drain and set aside, reserving 1/2 cup of pasta water.

In a large skillet, heat the extra virgin olive oil over medium heat. Add the minced garlic and red pepper flakes, and cook for 1-2 minutes until fragrant.

Add the shrimp to the skillet and cook for 2-3 minutes per side, or until pink and opaque.

Stir in the lemon zest and lemon juice, then add the cooked pasta to the skillet. Toss to coat the pasta evenly with the lemon garlic sauce.

If the sauce is too thick, add a splash of reserved pasta water to loosen it.

Season with salt and pepper to taste.

Garnish with chopped fresh parsley and serve hot.

Optionally, serve with grated Parmesan cheese on top.

Benefits:

This lemon garlic shrimp pasta is a light and flavorful dish that is rich in protein, fiber, and essential nutrients.

Shrimp is a low-calorie protein source that is high in heart-healthy omega-3 fatty acids and selenium.

Whole wheat pasta provides complex carbohydrates and fiber, which help maintain steady blood sugar levels and promote digestive health.

Cooking Time: 20 minutes

Recipe 24: Greek Turkey Burgers

Ingredients:

1 lb ground turkey

1/2 cup diced red onion

1/4 cup chopped fresh parsley

2 tablespoons chopped fresh mint

2 cloves garlic, minced

1 teaspoon dried oregano

1/2 teaspoon ground cumin

1/4 teaspoon paprika

Salt and pepper to taste

Whole wheat burger buns

Tzatziki sauce, lettuce, tomato, and red onion slices for serving

Instructions:

In a large mixing bowl, combine the ground turkey, diced red onion, chopped fresh parsley, chopped fresh mint, minced garlic, dried oregano, ground cumin, paprika, salt, and pepper. Mix until well combined.

Divide the turkey mixture into 4 equal portions and shape each portion into a burger patty.

Preheat grill or skillet over medium-high heat. Cook the turkey burgers for 4-5 minutes per side, or until cooked through and no longer pink in the center.

Toast the whole wheat burger buns on the grill or in a toaster.

Assemble the burgers by placing each turkey burger on a bun and topping with tzatziki sauce, lettuce, tomato, and red onion slices.

Serve hot with your favorite side dishes.

Benefits:

These Greek turkey burgers are a flavorful and nutritious alternative to traditional beef burgers.

Ground turkey is a lean protein source that is lower in saturated fat and cholesterol than beef.

Fresh herbs like parsley and mint add bright flavor and provide antioxidants and anti-inflammatory properties.

Cooking Time: 15 minutes

Recipe 25: Roasted Red Pepper and Lentil Soup

Ingredients:

1 cup dried red lentils, rinsed and drained

2 red bell peppers, roasted and diced

1 onion, diced

2 cloves garlic, minced

4 cups vegetable broth

1 teaspoon ground cumin

1/2 teaspoon smoked paprika

Salt and pepper to taste

Chopped fresh cilantro for garnish (optional)

Greek yogurt for serving (optional)

Instructions:

Preheat oven to 425°F (220°C). Place the whole red bell peppers on a baking sheet lined with parchment paper. Roast in the preheated oven for 25-30 minutes, or until the peppers are charred and tender.

Remove the peppers from the oven and transfer to a heatproof bowl. Cover with plastic wrap and let steam for 10 minutes.

Once cooled, peel off the skin of the peppers, remove the seeds and membranes, and dice the flesh.

In a large pot, heat olive oil over medium heat. Add the diced onion and minced garlic, and cook for 3-4 minutes until softened and fragrant.

Add the diced roasted red peppers, rinsed red lentils, vegetable broth, ground cumin, and smoked paprika to the pot. Stir to combine.

Bring the soup to a boil, then reduce the heat to low and simmer for 20-25 minutes, or until the lentils are tender.

Use an immersion blender to blend the soup until smooth and creamy. Alternatively, carefully transfer the soup to a blender and blend in batches until smooth.

Season with salt and pepper to taste.

Serve hot, garnished with chopped fresh cilantro and a dollop of Greek yogurt, if desired.

Benefits:

This roasted red pepper and lentil soup is a hearty and nutritious dish that is high in fiber, protein, and essential nutrients.

Red lentils are a good source of plant-based protein and fiber, which help promote satiety and stabilize blood sugar levels.

Red bell peppers are rich in vitamin C, antioxidants, and anti-inflammatory properties, which support immune health and cardiovascular health.

Cooking Time: 50 minutes

Recipe 26: Lemon Herb Quinoa Salad

Ingredients:

1 cup cooked quinoa

1 cup cherry tomatoes, halved

1/2 English cucumber, diced

1/4 cup sliced Kalamata olives

2 tablespoons chopped fresh parsley

2 tablespoons chopped fresh mint

2 tablespoons extra virgin olive oil

2 tablespoons fresh lemon juice

1 teaspoon lemon zest

Salt and pepper to taste

Crumbled feta cheese for garnish (optional)

Instructions:

In a large mixing bowl, combine the cooked quinoa, halved cherry tomatoes, diced cucumber, sliced Kalamata olives, chopped fresh parsley, and chopped fresh mint.

In a small bowl, whisk together the extra virgin olive oil, fresh lemon juice, lemon zest, salt, and pepper to make the dressing.

Pour the dressing over the quinoa salad ingredients and toss gently to coat.

Serve the lemon herb quinoa salad immediately, or refrigerate for 30 minutes to allow the flavors to meld.

Garnish with crumbled feta cheese before serving, if desired.

Benefits:

This lemon herb quinoa salad is a refreshing and nutritious dish that is high in fiber, protein, vitamins, and minerals.

Quinoa provides a complete source of protein and essential nutrients like fiber, potassium, and magnesium, which support cardiovascular health.

Fresh lemon juice and herbs like parsley and mint add vibrant flavor and provide antioxidants and anti-inflammatory properties.

Cooking Time: 15 minutes

Recipe 27: Mediterranean Stuffed Bell Peppers

Ingredients:

4 large bell peppers (any color)

1 cup cooked quinoa

1 cup diced tomatoes

1/2 cup diced cucumber

1/4 cup sliced Kalamata olives

1/4 cup crumbled feta cheese

2 tablespoons chopped fresh parsley

2 tablespoons extra virgin olive oil

1 tablespoon red wine vinegar

1 teaspoon dried oregano

Salt and pepper to taste

Lemon wedges for serving (optional)

Instructions:

Preheat oven to 375°F (190°C). Cut the tops off the bell peppers and remove the seeds and membranes.

In a large mixing bowl, combine the cooked quinoa, diced tomatoes, diced cucumber, sliced Kalamata olives, crumbled feta cheese, chopped fresh parsley, extra virgin olive oil, red wine vinegar, dried oregano, salt, and pepper.

Stuff each bell pepper with the quinoa mixture until they are filled to the top.

Place the stuffed bell peppers in a baking dish.

Cover the baking dish with aluminum foil and bake in the preheated oven for 30-35 minutes, or until the bell peppers are tender.

Remove from the oven and let cool for a few minutes before serving.

Serve the Mediterranean stuffed bell peppers hot with lemon wedges on the side, if desired.

Benefits:

These Mediterranean stuffed bell peppers are a flavorful and nutritious dish that is high in fiber, vitamins, and minerals.

Bell peppers are rich in antioxidants like vitamin C and beta-carotene, which support immune health and may help lower the risk of chronic diseases.

Quinoa provides plant-based protein and essential nutrients like fiber, which help promote satiety and stabilize blood sugar levels.

Cooking Time: 35 minutes

Recipe 28: Balsamic Glazed Chicken Breast

Ingredients:

4 boneless, skinless chicken breasts

1/4 cup balsamic vinegar

2 tablespoons honey or maple syrup

2 cloves garlic, minced

1 teaspoon dried thyme

Salt and pepper to taste

Fresh parsley for garnish

Instructions:

Preheat oven to 400°F (200°C). Line a baking dish with parchment paper.

In a small bowl, whisk together the balsamic vinegar, honey or maple syrup, minced garlic, dried thyme, salt, and pepper.

Place the chicken breasts in the prepared baking dish. Pour the balsamic glaze over the chicken, ensuring they are evenly coated.

Bake in the preheated oven for 20-25 minutes, or until the chicken is cooked through and no longer pink in the center.

Remove from the oven and let rest for a few minutes before serving.

Garnish with fresh parsley before serving.

Benefits:

This balsamic glazed chicken breast is a simple and flavorful dish that is high in protein and low in carbohydrates.

Balsamic vinegar adds a tangy flavor and provides antioxidants and potential blood sugar-regulating effects.

Chicken breast is a lean source of protein that is low in fat and calories, making it suitable for a healthy diet.

Cooking Time: 25 minutes

Recipe 29: Caprese Stuffed Portobello Mushrooms

Ingredients:

4 large Portobello mushrooms

2 large tomatoes, sliced

8 oz fresh mozzarella cheese, sliced

1/4 cup fresh basil leaves

2 tablespoons balsamic glaze

2 tablespoons extra virgin olive oil

Salt and pepper to taste

Instructions:

Preheat oven to 400°F (200°C). Line a baking sheet with parchment paper.

Remove the stems from the Portobello mushrooms and gently scrape out the gills with a spoon.

Brush both sides of the mushrooms with extra virgin olive oil and season with salt and pepper.

Place the mushrooms on the prepared baking sheet, gill side up.

Layer each mushroom with sliced tomatoes, fresh mozzarella cheese, and fresh basil leaves.

Drizzle balsamic glaze over the stuffed mushrooms.

Bake in the preheated oven for 15-20 minutes, or until the mushrooms are tender and the cheese is melted and bubbly.

Remove from the oven and let cool for a few minutes before serving.

Benefits:

These Caprese stuffed Portobello mushrooms are a flavorful and satisfying dish that is low in carbohydrates and rich in vitamins and minerals.

Portobello mushrooms are a good source of antioxidants, fiber, and essential nutrients like vitamin D and selenium.

Fresh tomatoes, mozzarella cheese, and basil provide a burst of flavor and additional nutrients like vitamin C, calcium, and potassium.

Cooking Time: 20 minutes

Recipe 30: Spicy Shrimp Stir-Fry

Ingredients:

1 lb large shrimp, peeled and deveined

2 tablespoons soy sauce (or tamari for gluten-free)

1 tablespoon Sriracha sauce (adjust to taste)

2 tablespoons hoisin sauce

1 tablespoon sesame oil

2 cloves garlic, minced

1 tablespoon grated ginger

2 cups mixed vegetables (bell peppers, broccoli, snap peas, carrots)

2 green onions, chopped

Cooked brown rice or cauliflower rice for serving

Instructions:

In a small bowl, whisk together the soy sauce, Sriracha sauce, hoisin sauce, and sesame oil to make the sauce. Set aside.

Heat a large skillet or wok over medium-high heat. Add a splash of oil and swirl to coat the pan.

Add the minced garlic and grated ginger to the skillet and stir-fry for 30 seconds, or until fragrant.

Add the mixed vegetables to the skillet and stir-fry for 3-4 minutes, or until crisp-tender.

Push the vegetables to one side of the skillet and add the shrimp to the other side. Cook the shrimp for 2-3 minutes per side, or until pink and opaque.

Pour the sauce over the shrimp and vegetables, tossing to coat evenly.

Cook for an additional 1-2 minutes, or until the sauce is heated through and slightly thickened.

Remove from the heat and sprinkle chopped green onions over the stir-fry.

Serve hot over cooked brown rice or cauliflower rice.

Benefits:

This spicy shrimp stir-fry is a quick and flavorful dish that is high in protein and packed with vegetables.

Shrimp is a low-calorie protein source that is rich in omega-3 fatty acids and selenium.

Mixed vegetables provide essential vitamins, minerals, and antioxidants, supporting overall health and immune function.

Cooking Time: 15 minutes

CONCLUSION

In conclusion, this High Blood Pressure Cookbook offers a diverse array of delicious and nutritious recipes designed to support a healthy lifestyle and manage hypertension. By emphasizing whole foods, lean proteins, healthy fats, and nutrient-dense ingredients, these recipes provide a balanced approach to cooking for optimal blood pressure management. From flavorful mains to satisfying sides and refreshing salads, each dish is carefully crafted to promote heart health while satisfying your taste buds.

With the principles, guidelines, and benefits outlined in this cookbook, along with the wide variety of recipes provided, you can embark on a culinary journey that not only supports your blood pressure goals but also inspires a lifelong commitment to wholesome eating. Whether you're seeking to lower your blood pressure or simply adopt a healthier diet, this cookbook serves as a valuable resource for nourishing your body and enhancing your overall well-being.

www.ingramcontent.com/pod-product-compliance
Lightning Source LLC
Chambersburg PA
CBHW050826250726
48653CB00006B/2455